CBD BOOK

A Beginners Guide to Understanding CBD including:

Symptoms of Structural, Emotional and Nutritional Stress

MARYANN STANGER ND

DISCLAIMER

This book is not a replacement for medical advice from a healthcare professional. The author and publisher do not dispense medical advice or prescribe the use of any technique as a form of treatment for physical, emotional or medical problems without the advice of a physician, either directly or indirectly. Application of information described herein is undertaken at the reader's risk, with no liability to the author or publisher. The contents of this book are for educational purposes only. Readers with medical concerns should consult with a healthcare professional.

CONTENTS

ACKNOWLEDGE

To each of you that have chosen to begin this journey to a healthier, happier self; I am excited to co-discover new hope and wholeness through the power of CBD. CBD is not a cure-all supplement, but it is showing great promise in a world grasping for hope in health. Through this compilation of research both science and anecdotal, it is my desire you find the education and relief of your symptoms for a healthier today and a better tomorrow.

Chapter One

Discovering CBD

Over the past 50 years, the public has become increasingly conscious of nutrition and its importance in our lives. Real interest began after WWII, when food supplements became available. Over the past 30 years, plant based supplements have grown into a multi-billion dollar industry.

When you enter the natural pharmacy of plant-based supplements, a whole world of possibilities may be waiting for you. Here you may find nature in one of its most powerful creations, CBD. CBD is an extract from the hemp plant's stems, blossoms and leaves. Worldwide, CBD is fast becoming a go-to for just about every age and just about every symptom. As new research is being uncovered on a daily basis, it's not just the plant-based pharmacy that is taking a hard look at the wonders of CBD. CBD can also be found at gas stations, coffee shops, drug stores, massage parlors, and even in fast food hamburgers. The FDA (Food and Drug Administration) is even recognizing its potential.

The Three Symptoms of Stress

As a Naturopathic Doctor, I've seen about everything there is to see when it comes to a disruption of health. I have used several brands of professional grade supplements in search of the perfect fix for hundreds of people and pets. But a symptom cannot be fixed if the root cause of the problem isn't addressed, and this is where CBD really steps up to the plate.

I estimate up to 90% of all symptoms begin with some form of stress. Symptoms are a sign that something is wrong in the body. Having symptoms does not necessarily mean a disease is present. Anytime a person has a symptom, looking at the internal environment will show us that some cell, tissue, or organ is under a considerable amount of stress. That stress may be *structural, emotional or nutritional.* All three stresses can result in the exact same symptom:

1. If you get in a car accident, you may receive a whiplash. You will my experience the *structural stress* of pain and inflammation.

2. Your boss calls and shocks you with the news that you have been fired. You may feel your neck lock up with the same pain and inflammation the person felt from a whiplash. This is considered an *emotional stress.*

3. You may love cake, but every time you eat it, you feel a pain in the back of your neck. You have never associated eating the cake with the pain in your neck, I mean, why would you? Because of your sensitivity to some ingredient in the cake, or a combination of ingredients, this may be causing a *nutritional stress* from a blockage in a meridian.

4. You have might have felt the knot in your stomach when you eat something that doesn't settle well and you may feel

a similar knot when you get bad news or get startled. This could be caused from *structural, emotional, nutritional stress or a combination of all three.*

The symptoms of stress do not stop with a pain in the neck or a knot in the stomach. The rest of the cells in the body will do what they can to maintain the internal environment. Some cells may even die trying. The body will rob Peter to pay Paul to keep the *whole body* alive and well. Thus symptoms became vast and far-reaching. The longer the stress is left unaddressed, the worse the symptoms become, even to the point of disease.

My CBD Discovery

I have tried about every natural pill, I have changed diets; I even created my own line of professional grade supplements, because I wanted my synergies to be powerful, effective at assisting people to better health. My goal was to offer everyone, within y reach, a better life. But getting to the heart of the stress was always the key to success when on that road to health. Although I made good dents in the symptoms of stress, I never found the ultimate results until I discovered CBD.

In 2017 I was introduced to CBD. I pushed it away because no way was I going encourage the use of 'marijuana'. As a law-abiding citizen I could not add marijuana to my practice in Idaho. Because I was curious how CBD worked and was willing to listen to the argument that "CBD was not marijuana", I began extensive research and I certainly was surprised what I found: CBD is not marijuana, the incredible effects CBD has within the body, the high percentage of people whose symptoms are altered by the use of CBD, the ease at which CBD can be administered, etc.

Shortly thereafter, I began using CBD to assist my family, my patients and about everyone that would give it a try: a veteran with 80% disability from war and suffering with severe PTSD, my 85 year old mother who cannot sleep at nights, a patient with anger issues, topically for an 87 year old man with bleeding thin skin, a grandmother with painful joints, a man with a rare form of bone cancer in his leg, many people with back pain and headaches, and more. Each person and each symptom was unique yet CBD seemed to assist in reducing the symptoms most every body. The symptoms of *structural, emotional and nutritional stress* began to dissipate.

Discovering CBD has blessed so many people in my circle of life. It would be a fairy tale ending if the story of CBD stopped here, but it doesn't. Because of the absolute incredible effects of CBD on the three stresses and because it is unregulated by the FDA, it has become a source of potential income for thousands of people around the world. This book is a guide for real people to understand and discover real CBD, the right way.

Chapter Two

CBD verses Marijuana

If you don't yet understand the differences between CBD and marijuana, this chapter will get you there.

CBD is an acronym for Cannabidiol. It's one of the 114 known cannabinoids found inside the cannabis plant; CBD, CBG CBN and THC are all cannabinoids, just to name a few. Yes, CBD can come from the same cannabis plant where marijuana (THC) is found. There are, however, significant differences between the two cannabinoids. The most important is the fact that CBD, unlike THC, is not . psychoactive. You cannot get 'high' from CBD. Psychoactive THC affects the mind or behavior and CBD will definitely not give you that same reaction of a high feeling, but it may affect your mind in positive ways.

> Hemp has been excluded from the Controlled Substances Act with the introduction of the 2018 Farm Bill.

CBD has been used in clinical trials for aiding seizure disorders, PTSD, anxiety, depression and a host of other symptoms. CBD is showing promise to aid in the direction of health and rejuvenation. With CBD, you can experience all the sought after health benefits of marijuana to a much larger scale and without the psychoactive effects.

Marijuana has increasingly become more potent in trahydrocannabinol (THC) over the past few decades as growers are cross breeding to get the THC content up to 30%. The results of this high THC are creating a marijuana that is causing addictions, more anxiety and less reduction of the three symptoms of stress.

As the THC percentage has increased in marijuana, the CBD content has naturally lowered, as there is only so much room inside a leaf or blossom.

The side effects of THC from marijuana can include the following symptoms:

- Dry mouth
- Dizziness or lightheadedness
- Dry red, itchy eyes
- Sleepiness and lethargy
- Euphoria or high
- Increased heart rate and blood pressure
- Increased appetite
- Paranoia

It is the CBD that contains most of the medicinal properties that assist with the symptoms of stress. In order for a cannabis plant to be legally classified as a hemp and not marijuana it must contain zero to .3% THC and no more.

Hemp verses Marijuana

Hemp is a cannabis plant that is harvested commercially for its seeds, stalks, leave and flowers. It can grow up to twenty feet. Cattle can safely graze in a hemp field.

Different parts of the plant have distinct uses: Seeds are used for hemp hearts, hemp oil, and hemp protein. These are high in vegan omegas. Stalks are a great source of fiber for building materials and clothing. Flowers and leaves are harvested for their cannabinoid (CBD) content. Hemp is also used for livestock feed.

Hemp has been excluded from the Controlled Substances Act with the introduction of the 2018 Farm Bill. According to the Farm Bill, hemp can be commercially grown and manufactured legally in the United States. Note here that state laws can override federal laws so the growing of hemp is, at the time of this publication, still illegal in 3 states.

On the other hand, Marijuana is harvested for its relaxing, and psychoactive properties. As opposed to hemp, the seeds and stalks of marijuana are not used commercially. Instead, the plant is cultivated for its highly resinous flowers containing an abundance of the cannabinoid, THC.

Marijuana is classified as a Schedule I substance under the Controlled Substances Act of 1970. Therefore, the US federal government doesn't recognize any medical uses of marijuana and claims it has a strong potential for abuse. Although marijuana remains federally illegal in the United States, some individual states have begun passing legislation that legalizes either medical or recreational marijuana use.

On the molecular level, CBD is the same whether it's found in hemp or marijuana plants. There are, however, several differences between CBD products. If you are consuming a USA organically grown, 3rd party lab tested CBD product, you never have to be concerned about the content of THC or the quality of the CBD. The only form of CBD that can currently be legally cultivated is hemp-derived CBD. This chart gives a visual to compare the hemp cannabis plant to the marijuana cannabis plant.

COMPARE	HEMP	MARIJUANA
FROM CANNABIS	Sativia	Indica or Sativa
THC% psychoactive cannibinoid	**Low THC** 0 - .3%	**High THC** 5 - 30%
CBD% relief of symptoms from stress	**High%** leaves, blossoms, stems	**Low%** blossoms
APPEARANCE	**Tall** slender, up to 20 feet	**Bushy** short, rounded bush
CLIMATE	**All Types** requires little water	**Humid** heat, rain fall, greenhouse
USES	**Nutritional** clothing, food, plastic rope, oil, medicinal...	**Recreational** some symptom relief mainly psychoactive effect

Currently, 47 states allow industrial hemp cultivation. This is a great thing for people who rely on CBD to assist the symptoms of their structural, emotional or nutritional stress.

Chapter Three

Every Body not Everybody

In my world as a Naturopathic Doctor, nutrition has traditionally been practiced through the recommendation of nutrients matched to the patient's symptoms. For example, if you have a cold, you take Vitamin C. If that doesn't work, add vitamins A and D or adrenal glandular support. If you are constipated, use a natural herbal laxative and change your diet. If that doesn't work, add magnesium and pancreatin with ox bile to assist digestion. These are natural pharmaceutical or magic bullet approaches that seek relief of the symptoms but they ignore the source of the problem.

While these applications have been successful to a certain degree for me, as a Naturopathic Doctor, they have not produced consistent results because such an approach fails to recognize the source of the individual stress symptom. No two bodies are alike. We have all been born with different genetic strengths and weaknesses, and the way we have treated our bodies has given us different states of vitality and recuperative capabilities.

You and a friend of yours may both be exhibiting symptoms of insomnia, but the source of stress causing the symptoms may be very different. Therefore, because each human body involved in the healing process cannot be generalized, a better system was needed. Instead of finding a remedy for a symptom that would benefit everybody (one word), I needed to concentrate on a unique solution for every body (two words), as every symptom in every body is a clinical story of its own.

Healing is an art as opposed to a science. A science teaches us to know and an art teaches us to do. Unless we use a comprehensive method of determining the struggle each body has

> Before you can understand CBD nutrition, you need to understand health and what disease is.

to maintain health, we cannot expect to address and correct the root cause of the stress symptom.

Everyone should know that a particular drug will help some bodies, will not be effective in other bodies, and may even harm still other bodies.

Before you can understand CBD nutrition, you need to understand health and what disease is. In the United States, only licensed health care professionals can treat disease and administer sick care. Fortunately, you do not need a license to practice nutrition and direct your own health care. You don't even need an education, or the ability to read and write, because every body eats.

Health is a normal condition of the body and mind, with all parts working normally while disease is a disturbed state of homeostasis. Disease comes with symptoms of stress, be it structural, emotional, nutritional or a combination of two or more.

If the symptoms are not addressed, then the body's response must continue to resist its effect and a state of compensation is reached. The part of the body affected by the stress symptom must then elicit aid from other tissues or, in most cases, begin using increased amounts of nutrients to maintain its heightened state of dysfunction. The situation will continue as long as the root cause of the stress is not addressed.

The body will eventually reach a state of exhaustion because of the fatigue on the affected tissues or organs. It is at this point where you can either move up towards health or down towards disease.

> **DISEASE**
>
> cannot be its own cause, nor can it be its own cure, and certainly not its own prevention

Medical research attempts to find magic bullets for each symptom, as if it were the primary problem. Painkillers, antacids, antidepressants, laxatives or surgery to remove the tissue or organ affected is most likely the medical go-to for treating the symptom.

If you view the body as a self-healing organism and understand that disease is disrupted health: it cannot be its own cause, nor can it be its own cure, and certainly not its own prevention, only then you can begin to grasp the very roots of how and why CBD works and its effects inside every body.

Chapter Four

How CBD Works

As a Naturopathic Doctor, this chapter is of most importance. All the hype about CBD and its miraculous benefits does not mean a thing if the anecdotal and scientific evidences are not there. Dr. Roger Adams and his team at the University of Illinois first discovered CBD in 1940. It wasn't until 1963 that real information and understanding on the power behind this hemp extract was beginning to come to light. Scientific and anecdotal research is now pouring in and showing CBD has a huge potential in the health industry.

CBD has been shown to: ease stress symptoms of anxiety, reduce pain and inflammation, and assist in preventing seizures, assist with sleep and many more. Because it is a natural extract, there are few, if any, side effects, but we will discuss those in chapter 5.

So how does CBD assist the body with so many symptoms of stress? CBD works with the body's endocannabinoid system, which is the system that regulates processes such as: pain, mood, appetite, and memory.

You may be wondering why you did not learn about the endocannabinoid system in school. It was first discovers in the 1990's by Dr. L.A. Matsuda. Scientists were trying to understand how THC from marijuana affected the body. What they discovered was an incredible, complex network of cannabinoid receptors in cells of both the central and peripheral nervous system.

We do not have a full and complete picture of what the ECS (Endocannabinoid System) does but we do know that the ECS helps fine-tune most of our vital physiological functions. It promotes homeostasis affecting everything from sleep, appetite, pain, inflammation, memory, mood, and even reproduction. So in basic terms, the ECS assists in the regulation of homeostasis across all major body systems ensuring that all systems work in harmony one with another.

CBD may assist self-healing in every body by encouraging the ECS to correct homeostasis…

Cannabinoid receptors are located through the body, however CB1 and CB2 are each better at receiving different cannabinoids than the other. For example, CB1 receptors, located primarily in the brain and central nervous system are more reactive to THC because of its psychoactive effect on the brain. CB2 receptors, located throughout the body, are more influenced by CBD. This is why CBD is often considered "non-psychoactive" because it does not react with the CB1 receptors found in the brain.

Experts believe CBD works by preventing endocannabinoids from being broken down. CBD increases levels of an endocannabinoid called anandamine, which creates anti-inflammatory effects through its activation of cannabinoid receptors.

Transient receptor potential (TRP) are other channels that affect the levels of calcium in cells. The action of CBD at these receptors may increase calcium levels in cells.

CBD also increases signaling of the 5HT-1A, a serotonin receptor. Serotonin assists the body in regulating mood balance. Serotonin system dysfunction is associated with depression and insomnia. The actions of CBD at serotonin receptors have been associated with decreasing anxiety as well.

In essence, CBD may assist in self-healing in every body by encouraging the ECS to correct homeostasis and by so doing begins the self-healing process. Although it appears as though CBD is just addressing the symptoms because relief may be felt with the first dose, in reality, it is assisting the body via the ECS to self-heal. Having said that, the relief of symptoms may not be an overnight process. CBD assists in the long processes of healing and as a positive side effect, makes the journey to health bearable.

In order to complete this journey, a proper diet must be included. Refined and processed foods should be avoided. A simple way to address diet is to purchase items with a single or a few ingredients. Spinach is an easy one as it contains spinach, a single ingredient. You should become a label reader. If you do not recognize an ingredient on the label, it most likely is a chemical food and not a food from nature. Avoiding these foods will aid your journey to health. With my patients, I used the 80% - 20% rule: 80% of the time, whole foods and no more than 20%

not-so-healthy foods. As disappointing as it is, pizza should be in the 20%.

With the discovery of the Endocannabinoid System and a beginning understanding on how it interacts and uses CBD, along with proper nutrition, you could very well be one step closer to a structural, emotional and nutritional stress-free life.

Chapter Five

The Safety of CBD

There were over 70,000 opioid related deaths in 2018. The total number of people that have died from overdosing on CBD is zero. As a Naturopathic Doctor and proponent of CBD, I have seen, first hand, how CBD assists in a wide variety of health issues. What I have not seen are negative side effects. Having said that, there are certainly people that may be sensitive to CBD and may even have a reaction. Although the side effects are extremely rare, here is a list of what most likely won't happen, but could in some bodies, both human and animals:

- Changes in mood
- Changes in appetite
- Diarrhea
- Dizziness
- Drowsiness
- Dry mouth
- Nausea
- Vomiting

> There were over 70,000 opioid related deaths in 2018. The total number of people that have died from overdosing on CBD is zero.

There's also some concern that the use of CBD may lead to increased levels of liver enzymes (a marker of liver damage or inflammation).

If you're considering trying CBD, it's important to discuss any potential side effects and adverse reactions with your physician. In one study, for instance, children with refractory epilepsy treated with CBD experienced an aggravation of seizures, sleepiness, digestive disturbances, and irritability. It was noted that the CBD they were taking contained trace amounts of THC. CBD with THC may impair your ability to drive safely or operate equipment and may have short- and long-term effects on your memory, attention, mood, heart rate, and mental health. If this is the case, CBD with the THC completely removed is available and the safest option to avoid any of these side effects.

CBD and Prescription Medication

Most prescription medications are metabolized in the liver by way of specific enzymes. One of the most important of these enzymes is a cytochrome P450 enzyme. They are critical in the metabolizing as much as 60% of drugs prescribed.

Some natural foods and/or supplements could alter the production of these enzymes. The result is that levels of certain drugs can build up in the blood increasing the drug effects, or in other cases, loose their effectiveness because they cannot be properly broken down.

The most well known example is grapefruit. In fact, the FDA has a list of medications that can interact with grapefruit.

Like grapefruit, CBD may temporarily inhibit certain cytochrome P450 enzymes.

How intensely this all plays out in your body mainly depends on the dosage of both the medication and the CBD that you're taking. If the concentration of CBD is high enough, it could inhibit the activity of enzymes, so you would get more out of the drug and into your system.

On the flip side, very low amounts of CBD don't seem to have that much of an effect on how well your body processes other medications. But unfortunately, there hasn't been enough research to determine how much CBD is considered non-interactive.

Other factors could also influence how CBD does or doesn't affect your medication. The timing of when you take both the medication(s) and CBD can also be a factor in how the drug may interact in your body.

Spacing out doses of medicine does help to reduce the workload on the liver. In other words, the risk of having a serious drug interaction may be lower if you take your medications and CBD at different times of the day. Check with your doctor for a list of possible drugs CBD may affect. Ultimately, how our body's process medication and the effect it will have, is heavily influenced by genetics, age and body size.

If you're unsure, it's always smart to talk to your physician before throwing CBD into the mix. If you're set on taking CBD, your doctor may be able to adjust the dose of your other medications. While CBD does seem relatively safe to use — and many people find it helps with their stress symptoms — you should be aware of any potential health risks.

Chapter Six

Understanding CBD Types

The four main types of CBD are full spectrum, broad spectrum, isolate and nano CBD. They simply refer to different ways CBD is processed and the final results of that production. There are benefits and drawbacks to all.

Full Spectrum refers to cannabis-derived from the leaves, stem and blossoms of the hemp plant. Full Spectrum contains CBD and other phytocannabionoids such as THC, CBN, CBG, and CBC. This type of CBD provides the 'entourage effect' as you getting all of the compounds together. In order to be classified as a legal CBD product, it must contain less that .3% THC and must be derived from the hemp plant and not the marijuana plant. Although at this level, and if a person takes only the recommended dosage, it is not likely they will test positive on a drug test for THC (marijuana). Currently, there are Full Spectrum CBD companies that have removed only the THC, making this full spectrum CBD legal in all 50 states. Only CBD that is backed by a 3rd party test showing the THC content, should be purchased.

There are 2 processes for extracting the Full Spectrum CBD from the hemp plant.

CO2 extraction uses supercritical carbon dioxide to separate the CBD oil from the plant material. During CO2 extraction, a series of pressurized chambers and pumps are used to expose CO2 to high pressure and very low temperatures, resulting in extracted oil containing high amounts of CBD.

Solvent extraction creates a resulting mixture of the CBD with the solvent. The solvent then evaporates, leaving pure CBD oil behind. Solvent extraction uses either hydrocarbons or natural solvents. The solvents used in hydrocarbon extraction (including naphtha, petroleum, butane, or propane) create concern. The solvent residue can be toxic and increase the cancer risk if they aren't fully eliminated during the evaporation step—which doesn't always happen. Some studies have found traces of petroleum or naphtha hydrocarbons residue in CBD products that used solvent extraction.

When the THC is removed from the Full Spectrum CBD it is often called **Broad Spectrum**. During the removal of THC for Broad Spectrum, often times other cannabinoids may also be removed or reduced.

CBD Isolate is a pure, crystalline powder that contains nearly 99% pure CBD. CBD isolate contains no other phytocannabionoids. All the plant matter contained in the hemp plant, including oils, waxes and chlorophyll, are removed. With a CBD isolate product, you not only miss the entourage effect with an isolate but you also miss the natural benefits of the synergy effect that comes from Full or Broad Spectrum.

Another emerging process in the CBD world is nanotechnology, often referred to as **Nano CBD**. Often used in beauty products, it focuses on breaking down compounds into 'nanoparticles.' This technology will continue to expand, as consumers make certain they are getting a high degree of results in the CBD products they consume and use topically. We did our own time lapsed research on CBD oil based soft gels vs Nano CBD soft gels. After 30 minutes the Nano CBD had broken down in the water while the oil based CBD soft gels were still in the shell. After 3 days, the oil based soft gels had yet to break down.

Bioavailability with results is what I look for when it comes to a CBD product. Currently, I recommend a Full Spectrum with zero THC that has been CO2 extracted and is make from USA, organically grown CBD with Nano CBD in a soft gel at a close second.

Chapter Seven

The Importance of Quality CBD

A year of schooling, multiple conferences, plus practicing as a Naturopathic Doctor have taught me many important things and at the top of my list is: read labels. Over half of the time, you will find chemicals and words too big to pronounce in what you expect to be a natural, product. So many so-called natural products contain fillers, additives and preservatives and CBD products are no exception to these added ingredients.

More often than not, what you see on the label is not what is inside the bottle. As an ND, I was so frustrated with all the 'natural' junk that I created my own line of quality, professional

> **6 Ps**
>
> 1. Professional Grade
> 2. Place of Origin
> 3. Purity _ "other ingredients"
> 4. Potency CBD mg per dose
> 5. Price per mg
> 6. People _ customer service

grade supplements and natural products with no fillers, no additives, and no artificial anything. I also made certain 3rd party tests came back to show what was on the label is what was in the bottle.

No matter how you take CBD, there are a few things you'll want to look for. I call these the 6 Ps of purchasing CBD products. Since the FDA does not currently regulate CBD products, it's important to ensure whatever you're buying has been lab-tested by a third party. This will allow you to see exactly what you're putting into your body, and verify that the product contains what the label says it does.

If the company does not have an website, an email address, a phone number and customer service person you can talk to, it may be a company you cannot trust to purchase your CBD products. Move on! There are legitimate companies and they can be easily found.

1. PROFESSIONAL GRADE – Full Spectrum CBD

Be sure to look for products made with full or broad-spectrum CBD that is C02 extracted — rather than distillate or isolate — with this you get the entourage effect and health benefits. Full spectrum products are less processed, which helps preserve some of cannabis's powerful organic compounds, like terpenes. (See Chapter 10 for more about Terpenes).

To be absolutely certain the CBD is of professional grade, always request 3rd party lab tests to verify the label matches the labs.

2. PLACE - U.S A. Organic Grown CBD

Look for products made from organic, United States grown

cannabis. Cannabis grown in the United States is subject to agricultural regulations and can't contain more than 0.3 percent THC. Organic ingredients mean you're less likely to consume pesticides or other chemicals.

3. PURITY -"Other Ingredients"

It is so important you read the label when purchasing a CBD product. Most CBD products contain fillers or other ingredients. Getting a 100% hemp product is critical in obtaining the best results for both the effects of the CBD and the benefits for your health. Make certain what you purchase is 100% pure cannabis full spectrum CBD hemp and contains: no artificial colors or flavors, no fillers, and no additives.

4. POTENCY - Dosage of CBD mg per serving

This is a very grey area and can be so confusing. You can look on Amazon.com and find bottles of Hemp Oil claiming to have 80,000 mg of 'Hemp Extract' aka CBD Oil.   This is virtually impossible as 1 oz. can only have 28,000 milligrams at maximum of anything.

If you were to purchase 28,000 mg of pure CBD oil, it would cost you well over $1,000.

A legitimate CBD oil company will have the mg of the CBD listed on their label and will back this with 3rd party lab testing.

When purchasing CBD (Hemp Extract or Premium Hemp

or Hemp Oil) on 3rd party sites such as Amazon, most of the sellers are either using cheap, poor quality CBD or they contain no CBD oil at all.

If it is a legitimate company they will have a website and 3rd party lab tests. Make certain your CBD products meet the 6 Ps.

5. PRICE – Quality Matters

Again, the company is critical when it comes to price. 300 mg of CBD in a base of one oz. hemp oil is a good starting point for a real CBD company. This will equal about ten milligrams of pure, full spectrum CBD per serving. This could sell between $25-$80 if it is a legitimate CBD product. The higher price does not make it a higher quality product. It is just a company that wants to make more money or it is a multi-level (MLM) company that will be paying several people a piece of that bottle's selling price.

A stronger dose of CBD could be as high as fifty milligrams per serving. This is very costly and you should expect to pay upwards of $10 per dose. A one-ounce bottle of 50 milligrams per serving might range between $100-$300.

6. People – Customer Service

Does the CBD company a website? An email address? A phone number? When you call the phone number do you speak to a recording or a real person? Does the CBD company offer any educational information? Real people are a very important part of determining if your CBD product will be a high quality product.

Give them a call and see who answers.

Looking for the **6 Ps** before purchasing any CBD product will inevitably save you precious time and money plus it will ensure you receive a product that will be effective in aiding you on your journey towards a symptom-free life.

Chapter Eight

Pregnancy, Children and CBD

Being a mother of 8, I can honestly say pregnancy can be both a beautiful and miserable few months. Most expecting mothers experience symptoms of stress, be it structural, emotional, nutritional or a combination of all three. Cramping, insomnia, anxiety, morning sickness, and many more are just a few of the stress symptoms that occur throughout pregnancy.

CBD had been shown to support many of these stress symptoms. It is critical to purchase CBD that is THC-free. Not only can THC be harmful for the expecting mother it can also cause problems with the baby. Always check with your doctor first and require 3rd party tests to verify the THC content before purchasing any CBD product.

CBD for Children

Increasingly, parents are turning to CBD: anger issues, emotional distress, seizures, ADHD, etc. Some parents even say giving their child CBD has helped with autism and seizure disorders. CBD for seizures in children and adults has had extensive research. CBD is being used to assist seizure disorders. On a federal level, the FDA has approved a CBD drug to assist with seizure disorders.

If you're wondering whether CBD could help your child, find someone knowledgeable to consult. You should check with your child's doctor noting that in some cases, the CBD may interact with certain medications. There are many doctors not educated in the use of CBD for various conditions in kids so you may need to broaden your search. You can look for a ND (Naturopathic Doctor) in your area as they are becoming more common and may have the knowledge of CBD for children.

Though there are some topical treatments, and they are highly recommended for topical needs, CBD is typically administered orally to children. Emerging research shows there can be incredible benefits for children with few and rare side effects.

The most common negative side effects of CBD on children are drowsiness and dry mouth, but these often go away after a couple of weeks. Overdosing with CBD might only take place if the CBD product contains even trace amounts of THC.

Overdosing may give the appearance of your child being high. Depending on how significantly a child has been overdosed, the effects of that can be long lasting, even days. If you suspect an overdose, take your child to the hospital immediately. This is one of several reasons it is essential you only use a CBD that is 3rd party lab tested to be THC-free and to speak with a professional before administering CBD to anyone under the age of 18.

THC-free and the correct dosage are both imperative when giving CBD to children. As is the case with any supplement, if your child is under the care of a doctor, especially if your child is taking any medication, you should visit with him/her before giving CBD to anyone under 18 years of age.

Success for children has everything to do with dosing. Your child's body weight, age and symptoms will determine the amount that should be given to your child. It is never recommended to go above the suggested dosage found on the bottles label, unless advised by a medical professional.

Children seem to gravitate to the gummies and flavored CBD oils. Make certain both are pure, do not contain fillers or additives and large amounts of sugar.

CBD can be pricey because of the cost in growing the plants and extracting the oil so make certain what you are giving your child has been 3rd party tested.

Dosages for children under age 5 should only be given under the direction of a doctor's care, as well as any child on medication.

If a child is 10 years of age or less, starting dosage could be 2 milligrams of CBD, twice daily. Children between the age of 10-17 and weighing less than 100 lbs. could start at 4 mg twice daily. If a child over 10 years of age weighs 100 lbs. or more, they could begin with 5 mg twice daily. The dose could increase until stress symptoms have been reduced.

Again, consult a professional before giving any CBD to a child under the age of 18, especially if the child is on medication.

Chapter Nine

CBD for Pets

I wish you could meet my sweet puppy, Guess. I never thought I would be a pet owner because with 8 children, I had plenty to do. Now the children are grown and I find myself with a toy poodle.

Sundays at my house are crazy. After attending church, all 8 children with their spouses and my 28 grandchildren make their way to grandmas for a nutritious home cooked meal. To say the least, this many people can put Guess into overdrive and overwhelm. Giving him a CBD dog treat about an hour before the gang of up to 40 people arrive, allows him to calmly enjoy the few hours of commotion. It also calms me because I do not have to worrying about his stress level.

While there's no definitive scientific data on using CBD to help your pets, there is plenty of anecdotal evidence from hundreds of pet owners suggesting it can assist pain, especially neuropathic pain, as well as helping to control seizures. As noted above, it is also extremely helpful in assisting hyperactive, agitated or aggressive pets.

There are a possible few rare side effects:

- Dry mouth: Research has shown that CBD can decrease the production of saliva. For animals, this would manifest as an increased thirst.

- Lowered blood pressure: High doses of CBD have been known to cause a temporary drop in blood pressure. Even though the drop is small, it might create a brief feeling of light-headedness.

- Drowsiness: Pet owners have used CBD to treat anxiety. The calming effect of CBD can also cause slight drowsiness, especially when using higher doses.

The safety and risks of using CBD for animals have yet to be researched. If you decide to try CBD for your pet, there are a few things to keep in mind. Not all CBD is the same; you'll want a high-quality USA organically grown CBD. This will allow your pet to not only have a safe CBD but also a more effective product for your money, as real CBD is not cheap. A cheaper option could have toxic substances such as pesticides, herbicides, or heavy metals and may actually contain zero CBD. Make sure your CBD is free of additives by requesting a 3rd party lab test. You will also want to make sure there is no THC in the product as THC can have a severe negative affect on pets.

You can buy pet treats containing CBD, but the best form to administer is an oil or tincture. This way, you can adjust your pet's dose drop by drop. If you do buy the CBD treats, make certain they are veterinarian formulated.

CBD is available in many convenient forms. Extracts can

be given from a dropper bottle directly into the mouth, added to food, dropped on a treat, rubbed into bare skin or inside the ears, or dropped on an animal's paw so they will lick it off. You can also find hemp CBD treats, hemp CBD gel caps, and topical hemp CBD ointments.

Dosage can vary quite a bit from one situation to the next. It may be necessary to experiment a little to find the right amount, and how often to give.

Typical suggested starting dose: 1 mg – 5 mg per 10 lbs. of bodyweight. Start with a dose on the low end of the range. Changes usually occur within 30 minutes. If there is no change after an hour, increase the dosage. Occasionally improvements will take more than one treatment. To control pain, give approximately every 8 hours. For other uses, or to break unwanted behavior patterns, give up to three times daily.

Look for CBD products for dogs, cats and horses that are made from a concentrated extract of cannabidiol (CBD) in a base of virgin hemp oil. The CBD should be obtained by the CO2 extraction method for a clean solvent-free extract. The whole hemp plant should be used to produce a full spectrum extract with hundreds of trace compounds for the entourage effect.

Overdosing with CBD might only take place if the CBD product contains even trace amounts of THC. This is one of several reasons it is essential you only use a CBD that is 3rd party lab tested to be THC-free.

Life-threatening risks for pets from CBD are rare and

usually only occur if the quality of the CBD is poor or if it contains THC. Toxicity more often occurs when a pet has eaten a product that contains chocolate, coffee, or raisins. Even if the THC toxicity is not excessive, they can sometimes have problems due to other ingredients. This is another reason it is important to get a product that is 100% pure hemp, as many current CBD products contain fillers such as MCT or olive oil, artificial flavors or sweeteners.

CBD FOR DOGS –

CBD can be used to assist seizures, nausea, stress, anxiety, joint disorders, back pain, symptoms of cancer, and gastrointestinal issues, among other health conditions in dogs.

Relief is provided as CBD interacts with the endocannabinoid system. Unlike some traditional pain medicine for dogs, THC-free CBD has no known life-threatening side effects with proper dosage.

CBD FOR CATS

CBD has been shown to have anti-inflammatory properties, aid with joint health, reduce anxiety, improve overall well being, reduce pain and lessen or eliminate seizure activity. Topically it can assist with many concerns as well.

CBD FOR HORSES

From first-hand accounts of horse owners, hemp-derived CBD appears to stimulate the horse's ECS in the same way it does yours. It is well tolerated, without any euphoric or adverse effects.

Chapter Ten

CBD and Aromatherapy

Aromatherapy has become very popular in recent years. As a certified aromatherapist, I understand the profound effect the sense of smell can have on the stresses of structure, emotion and nutrition. Have you ever smelled an aroma and said to yourself, "that reminds me of my grandma's house when I was little"? It creates a fond memory as you close your eyes and take another whiff. It can give you a sense of belonging and comfort. Someone else in the room may state that it stinks because they lack the experience with the aroma that you have.

So the question is what really happens when you stop to smell a rose? Aromas are made of terpenes from plants. When you inhale the aroma of a rose, you're actually inhaling molecules or terpenes that the rose releases into the air. Terpenes are what give an orange its citrusy smell. They give pine trees their unique aroma. They're even responsible for the relaxing effects of lavender. Terpenes are the molecules that determine how things smell.

So far in this book, we have learned that cannabinoids are the compounds in the cannabis plant that work with the body to encourage a reduction in the symptoms of stress and, as science is showing, may promote healing with the endocannabinoid system. It is also coming to light that cannabis terpenes can play a big role on your journey to health as well. In fact, cannabinoids and terpenes work together in synergy to create an entourage effect.

It's the whole plant that does the best job, not just isolated CBD. While relief does come from using isolated CBD, whole plant therapy goes beyond the relief of symptoms and moves into the realm of healing. And ultimately, isn't that what we are longing for, relief of symptoms and healing?

As an aromatherapist, I have seen the benefits of various essential oils and their use to provide relief of the symptoms of structural, emotional and nutritional stress by aroma, topically, and other methods. CBD has gained popularity for its various uses such as: to ease pain and inflammation, improve mood and sleep, and even provide relief for your pets. Because CBD contains powerfully effective terpenes, why not include it in a blend with other essential oils that may also contain soothing and healing terpenes?

Currently, there are over 20,000 terpenes known and the cannabis plant has more than 100 of these terpenes. I find this to be very interesting and telling as to why cannabis can be beneficial just by it's aroma alone.

Terpenes may vary significantly in each hemp plant. If terpenes are of importance to you, look at the 3rd party lab tests from your CBD seller. The terpenes available in that product should be listed on the test. If none are listed, it may be an isolate that contains no terpenes.

Here are a few terpenes in the cannabis plant and elsewhere in nature. Also included is the possible effect they have on the symptoms of structural, emotional and nutritional stress:

Myrcene, which can also be found in mangoes, is the primary terpene found in cannabis plants. In fact, up to 65 percent of its terpene profile could be myrcene. Myrcene is responsible for giving cannabis its distinctive aroma. Myrcene has relaxing properties as well as anti-inflammatory properties.

The second most abundant terpene found in cannabis is **limonene.** It is also found in citrus fruits and is responsible for the citrusy smell. Limonene has powerful anti-fungal and anti-bacterial properties. Its great smell makes it a common additive in household cleaning and cosmetic products. Limonene has been shown to assist in the reduction of structural, emotional and nutritional stress. Adding a few drops of lemon EO with CBD can assist in soothing the digestive system. Diffusing the same blend could boost a mood.

Pinene is found in the pine tree and is what gives pine needles its incredible aroma. Pinene is can positively affect the bronchia, but also has strong anti-inflammatory and antiseptic properties that have been used for centuries in herbal medicines.

Lavender is the most used of all essential oils. If you have used lavender then you are familiar with the aroma of the terpene **linalool**. Linalool is known for the stress-relieving, anti-anxiety, and anti-depressant effects. Linalool can lift you or calm you; therefore it is a perfect terpene for both anxiety and depression.

Caryophyllene is a terpene, which has a spicy, woody, peppery scent. This terpene is also found in black pepper and cinnamon. Studies show this terpene is capable of performing a lot of jobs including the fight against: anxiety, depression, and inflammation.

Beta-Gamma-Eudesmol is found in rosemary and thyme. This terpene may have a toxic effect on cancer cells.

Guaiol found in tropical hardwoods, such as cypress trees. It is most known for having anti-inflammatory properties, as well as antioxidant properties.

Beta-Eudesmol found in walnut and basil. It has antioxidant and contains antimicrobial properties.

When you combine the benefits of essential oil aromatherapy and the terpene benefits of CBD, symptom relief may become even more possible. Why stop with only the ingestion of CBD when you could also benefit immensely with the aroma, in combination with other essential oils?

A line of pure, undiluted CBD, infused with the highest quality of essential oils, as individual or as a synergy, may increase the benefits of your regular essential oil use and add to the benefits of CBD ingestion. It appears to be a win/win for every body.

Chapter Eleven

CBD and Stress Symptoms

As a Naturopathic Doctor, I have much anecdotal research concerning CBD and it's effect on symptoms. My personal and professional belief is that CBD is one of the greatest natural finds in the history of mankind. It is not a cure-all or a fix-all but it has been shown to be incredible effective as a symptom reducer, and because of the interaction with the Endocannabinoid System, CBD may assist in the symptom relief caused from structural, emotional and nutritional stress.

Anxiety

CBD is commonly used to assist with the stress of **anxiety**. Anxiety could be a result of structural, emotional or nutritional stress or a combination. Anxiety can also be genetically enhanced. Finding the root cause of the anxiety can be a difficult task. If you look back to when the symptom of anxiety first occurred, you may be able to associate it with an accident, an emotional event or a food that acerbated the symptom. CBD aids in relaxation, making it a popular alternative treatment for assisting mood disorders such as anxiety.

Depression

Almost 17% of the population struggles with some symptoms of **depression**. It's more common in women than men. A growing number of people are using CBD products to assist in reducing the symptoms of depression. Like depressed people, chronic users of THC tend to have a smaller hippocampus, but CBD helps prevent this shrinking. Avoiding CBD products with even a trace of THC is critical for people suffering with depression. Smaller doses of CBD may affect depression more than larger doses, but this can be very different for every body. Start small and work up until the CBD is assisting your symptoms.

Pain

An entire book could be written on the symptom of **pain**. Each and every one of us has most likely experienced the symptom of pain structurally as in a sprained ankle, a smashed finger, a broken bone or an inflamed joint. We have most likely all encountered emotional pain from the loss of a loved one, divorce, an argument, a problem at work, a difficult child, and the list goes on and on. Nutritionally, more than likely, we have also experienced pain: heart burn, indigestion, diarrhea, nausea, constipation and more.

Both the acute and chronic symptoms of pain have been greatly assisted by the use of CBD products, topically and internally. You don't have to look far to find someone that can testify about CBD and his or her reduction or removal of the symptom of pain.

In order to fully understand CBD and its incredible effect on pain, we need to go inside the body's endocannabinoid system and look at the receptor CB2. The CB2 receptors can be found throughout the body including in the immune system. This makes them more responsible for the body's response to pain and inflammation. CBD impacts the CB2 receptors. And it does so indirectly, not by attaching to the CB2 receptor, but by encouraging the body to make more of its own cannabinoids. This creates a positive effect on the body's pain and inflammation response. CBD might even help the body heal itself. It isn't like a drug that tricks the brain into thinking the pain is gone, CBD actually helps the body fix the cause of the symptom and doesn't just cover it up.

Inflammation

Pain cannot be mentioned without discussing **inflammation** as the two go hand in hand. Inflammation primarily causes pain because the swelling pushes against sensitive nerve endings. This sends signals to the brain. People will feel the symptoms of pain, stiffness, discomfort, distress, and even agony, depending on the severity of the inflammation. CBD is being heavily studied for its anti-inflammatory properties.

Sleep

CBD may play an important role in **sleep**. The terpene

myrcene, which is the prominent terpene in CBD, acts as a natural sedative and improves the speed of falling to sleep and the quality of sleep. A good night's sleep assists with body repair, better cognition, and increased immunity. Preliminary research into cannabis and insomnia suggests that CBD may have therapeutic potential for the assisting insomnia. CBD may hold promise for REM sleep as well. Scientific research on CBD and sleep is just beginning, but the anecdotal evidence is overwhelming. Lower doses of CBD can have a lift or wake up effect, while larger doses tend to be more of a sedative for a better sleep. This can vary greatly, so it is best to experiment to make certain it is what you need for better nights sleep.

Skin

Topically, CBD can assist with many **skin problems**. It is a natural alternative to steroid cream, but unless directed by a doctor, should not replace any prescribed medication, even a topical prescription.

CBD has an anti-inflammatory effect on the skin and body. CBD also soothes itchiness and redness, two of the more prominent problems of the skin symptoms of stress. Be cautious when selecting a CBD topical to make certain the CBD content is as claimed on label and the other ingredients will assist in the healing and not cause further harm.

Chapter Twelve

Purchasing CBD

It's estimated that by 2020, the consumer market for CBD products will reach over two billion dollars. CBD is popping up everywhere including: fast food chains, grocery stores, gas stations, drug store, coffee shops, spas, 3rd party websites such as eBay, Wal-Mart and Amazon, and countless other websites from around the world. So, where and how do you find a reputable company with a quality product?

I am a Naturopathic Doctor and founder of Zatural.com. Years before CBD became a popular answer to so many stresses, Zatural was selling the absolute highest quality hemp seed oil on the market. We were getting it on a monthly basis from an organic farm in Canada, so it was the ultimate of fresh. At first it was selling slow as many people thought hemp was marijuana. Then as knowledge began to grow that hemp and marijuana were not the same plant and people began learning the benefits of hemp oil for health, the sale of our hemp seed products exploded. We were selling as many as 50,000 bottles a month in varies sizes on Amazon alone. Our most popular size of hemp seed oil was 16 oz. for $19.99.

3rd party websites such as Amazon, EBay, Wal-Mart, etc. do not allow the sale of CBD so when people were using the search term "CBD oil" they would be directed to our hemp oil because we were the number one selling hemp oil.

People then began purchasing our hemp seed oil, thinking it was CBD because that's where their search sent them. The customer would then complain to Amazon that we were misrepresenting our product as a CBD product. In response to the complaints, our hemp oil was removed from Amazon. We worked through that and were finally able to get our hemp oil for sale on Amazon again.

Over time we noticed a significant decrease in our hemp oil sales. Taking the number one spot on Amazon under the search terms of 'hemp oil' or 'CBD Oil' was no longer our 16 oz. bottle of fresh, pure hemp seed oil at $19.99, but it was now a 1 oz. bottle of 'hemp extract' for $29.99. Hemp extract is, in most cases, actually CBD, incognito for 3rd party sites such as Amazon that don't allow the sell of CBD products.

This became another huge problem as nowhere on the label can you list the CBD amount in a bottle, so instead, the label might say something like "1000 mg Hemp Oil". Consumers were going crazy over this, thinking they were getting 1000 milligrams of CBD for only $29.99 when in reality, no one knows what amount of CBD if any, was in the bottle of Hemp Extract, possibly not even the manufacturer.

70% of the bottles of 'hemp extract" sold on 3rd party sites were tested and found to contain zero CBD. Not only did they not contain CBD, but also many contain bacteria, fillers or harmful compounds not listed on the label.

This problem has recently become worse. Amazon caught on and started attempting to control the hemp extract. They said they now only allow hemp oil to be sold and no longer hemp extract. So what did companies do? They simple changed the label from Hemp Extract to Hemp Oil. Now if you search "CBD oil" or "hemp oil" on amazon you will see one-ounce bottles of hemp oil that contain 80,000 milligrams or more for $9.99. Uneducated consumers love the fact that they can get 80,000 mg of CBD for only $9.99. Not only do they think this product has 80,000 mg of CBD, but it also has over 4,000, 5 star reviews so it has to be real and fantastic, right?

There can only be, at the most, 28,000 milligrams in a fluid ounce, so any more than 28,000 mg is a huge red flag. 28,000 mg of pure full spectrum CBD would be over $1,000, not $9.99.

The purpose in telling you this story is to let you know there are a lot of bad CBD companies that care nothing about the health of their customers. For the consumer, it can be tough to know where and what to buy.

So here is my advice in a nutshell and I will start with the most popular way to buy CBD, online.

Buying CBD **online** has its perks: it's convenient, easy to do, has the best prices and offers the widest range of products in virtually every category available. Many sites offer fast, free shipping to all 50 states, making it easier for consumers who don't have access to brick-and-mortar stores or cannot afford the high prices they require because the overhead expenses of a building and employees have to be added into the cost of their CBD products.

Just like my Amazon story above, you never know if the product you are receiving even contains CBD, whether in a storefront or online. My advice is to only purchase CBD from a company that has a website, an email address and a customer service phone number where you can talk to a real person. Buying CBD (or hemp oil) products on any 3rd party site is a risk and could ultimately be harmful to your health and your pocketbook unless you are certain it is a legitimate company and follows the 6 Ps (see Chapter 7).

Even Zatural sells hemp oil products on 3rd party websites and they are of the upmost quality. But the only way you personally could know that is to research Zatural.

- Do they have a phone number?
- Do they have a website?
- Do you talk to a real person when you call that phone number?
- Do they have 3rd party lab tests?
- Do they have free returns?
- Are they made from USA organically grown CBD?

Many states where the sale of marijuana is legal, have establishments which once focused almost entirely on marijuana products, are now seeing a demand for CBD and are providing products to meet that demand.

The same principle applies to the products purchased from these stores as it does to online shopping. Ask for 3rd party lab tests. Does the brand you are purchasing have a website? Do they have a customer service phone number?

Many **chain stores** are private labeling the CBD they carry on their shelf. This can be tricky as they are reaching out to other companies to do the manufacturing of their CBD line. In this case, it is difficult to know if their CBD products have been 3rd party tested for label accuracy or if it contains any CBD at all.

There are also **MLM** (multi level marketing) CBD companies claiming you will need to purchase their product in order to get the best CBD. Their prices reflect the multi level thinking because many people get a cut from the sell price of one bottle, the ultimate price of that product will increase. MLM CBD products usually cost twice as much or more as other reputable companies.

Here is a list of the top MLM CBD companies:

- Kannaway
- Hemp Herbals
- HempWorx
- Dose of Nature
- Bocannaco

When purchasing quality CBD products from a reputable company it is still critical to read the ingredients. Because of the cost of pure, full spectrum CBD, most companies, even reputable ones, do all they can to control their bottom line of profits. Some of the leading sellers of CBD oil put the CBD in a base of MCT oil, olive oil or another oil. MCT Oil is much cheaper than pure, organically grown hemp oil. MCT oil is derived from palm kernels through a chemical process. MCT oil never expires, so it can be 10 years old and still used in the product as fresh oil.

Hemp oil has a shelf life of 18 months, if kept in a cool dark place. That makes it harder to mass-produce and mass-production saves the manufacturer money.

Even though the synergy of hemp seed oil with the CBD extract is the ultimate synergy for your journey to health, for most companies it's about the bottom line, not the consumer's health.

Two of China's regions are quietly leading the boom of cultivating cannabis to produce CBD. The fact that most CBD in products sold in the United States are coming from overseas and are completely unregulated is a scary thought. If your CBD doesn't state it is grown organically in the USA, then it most likely is not and almost certainly is an inferior CBD. Right now the CBD boom around the world is more about the money than about your well-being.

Add to that the animal gelatin and artificial ingredients found in many reputable CBD products, along with preservatives and other fillers. Seems ironic to me to take CBD for your health when it is filled with ingredients that are not good for you.

High quality CBD is expensive. Pure, USA organically grown CBD wholesale pricing currently start around $10,000 per kilogram. That is why the price on the shelf can exceed $200 for a

1 oz. bottle, if the CBD milligram is high.

The CBD mg is also important and can be quite confusing. You might think you are purchasing a one-ounce bottle of CO_2 extracted, 300 mg of "pure CBD Oil". Further label reading shows the 300 milligrams is actually the milligrams of the full hemp extract and not the CBD. The true CBD milligram may be 30 for the entire bottle, not per serving.

One of the most reputable and highest selling CBD company's is a great example of money over well-being. This company does not state the place their CBD is grown. With a little investigation I found it is not from the USA at all and the country source of their CBD changes, based on price and availability.

One of this company's highest selling CBD oils shows just how confusing a label can be. It states: The hemp oil (from the aerial plant) per serving _13 milligrams. In smaller print it explains: only 3 mg of the 13 mg is CBD. Under 'other ingredients' the first ingredient is olive oil with monk fruit, silica, monolaurin, quillaja saponaria, ascorbyl palmitate, alpha tocopherol, and water. Really? I get the shelf life of this product can last for a very long time, but shouldn't the consumer of CBD oil want or demand fresh CBD products that are not filled with unhealthy ingredients? On top of all this the CBD they sell is also quite expensive. Remember the 6 Ps!

A good CBD oil should have 2 ingredients: Hemp Oil as a base and Full Spectrum CBD ectract, with our without the legal amount of THC which is less than 0.3%. It should be CO_2

extracted from USA organically grown Hemp. If flavors are added they should be of natural origin. If a sweetener is added it should be stevia or monk fruit only. So at tops, the best CBD oil should have a simple label with 2-4 natural ingredients.

A good CBD company should have 3rd party lab tests showing the cannabinoids and the terpenes in their ingestible products. This is critical because of the THC content. To be legal in every state the CBD product must be THC-free which makes it safe for all ages and pets.

A good CBD company should be GMP compliant. This is an FDA requirement for all supplements or ingestible food product. It stands for Good Manufacturing Practice. The requirements are steep and expensive for a company to implement, but it assures the sanitation of the manufacturing facility and the quality of the ingredients. Plus it ensures what is on the label is actually what is in the bottle.

This chapter may concern you about purchasing any CBD product, and for good reason, but there are GMP compliant, 6 Ps companies out there. Do your research and you will find the perfect company for your CBD needs.

Chapter Thirteen

Ways to Take CBD

CBD can be a delicious gummy or a dreaded dropper. Each method comes with its perks. While CBD has a variety of uses, some forms of CBD are more bioavailable than others. This means the body more readily absorbs them. This chapter will help you navigate each method of CBD consumption, and figure out what might work best to assist your symptoms of stress.

Edibles are a great way to try CBD. You can find a variety of CBD edibles including gummies, chocolate and more. Edibles are subject to something called the first pass effect. During the first pass effect, CBD is partially broken down by the liver and in the digestive tract. This means that the effects of CBD can take up to two hours to kick in, and you'll absorb only 20 to 30 percent of the CBD you consumed. Edibles may also be filled with artificial colors, flavors and/or corn syrup and other harmful sugars, preservatives and ingredients. Make certain if you are taking CBD for health benefits you are not consuming edibles that contain harmful ingredients. Find a company where the gummies are 100% organic, vegan with natural colors and flavors and are high in CBD mg (20mg per gummy). Edibles are a delicious option for the elderly and children and anyone else that cannot take pills or doesn't like to take drops.

Sublingual is designed to be absorbed under your tongue. The best CBD is CO_2 extracted. Letting the product absorb under your tongue rather than subjecting it to the digestive tract preserves more of the CBD milligrams, and you'll feel results faster plus it may be easier on the liver.

Choose sublingual if you're looking for quicker results and a higher yield from the CBD milligram bioavailability. With sublingual's it is also important to read the label. Many sublinguals contain ingredients and fillers such as MCT oil, coconut oil, olive oil, sugar, artificial ingredients and/or preservatives. Find a company where the sublingual's are 100% pure hemp and contain the highest USA organically grown CBD milligram for your dollar.

Soft gels are a great alternative to the drops. They usually contain 10, 15 or 25 milligrams but may go up to 100 mg of CBD. They are available in a Nano CBD or an oil based CBD. The Nano CBD absorbs quicker into the system and may be easier on the liver. Nano may allow the body to access more milligrams of CBD per serving. Additional herbs such as turmeric for pain and inflammation or melatonin for sleep assistance can be added to the soft gel for additional benefits.

CBD **topicals** can be applied directly to the skin. You can find CBD-infused lotions, balms, creams, salves, and even patches. Topicals are a great choice when it comes to assisting localized pain or skin conditions.

Using a product that contains additional analgesics such as menthol, camphor and capsaicin may bring even more therapeutic potential.

The permeability of your skin is pretty poor relative to mucous membranes, like sublingual tissue. That means when using a topical product, you'll want to choose one with a high amount of CBD and apply it generously. A good starting point of topical is 250 mg of CBD per ounce of product.

You can **vape** CBD using a vaporizer with a cartridge that contains CBD oil, or even inhale CBD concentrates such as sugar waxes with any vape pen that has a chamber for concentrates.

Vaping and smoking allow the CBD to go directly into your bloodstream, so you'll feel effects much faster than you will with other methods. With vaping, the verdict is still out on how safe it is, so it may not be the best choice.

If you do decide to vape, avoid CBD vape cartridges made with thinning agents or carriers such as fractionated coconut oil (MCT), propylene glycol, or vegetable glycerin. These have been found to be dangerous and could damage the lung tissue.

Before vaping CBD, you should also talk to your doctor, especially if you're currently on any medication.

Whether you choose edible, sublingual, soft gel, topical, a CBD infused essential oil or a combination of the above, the benefits of CBD may quickly change your level of stress be it structural, emotional or nutritional.

Chapter Fourteen

CBD Dosage

Every body is different, and each person may require a different amount of CBD to receive the therapeutic benefits they are searching for. Let me share, through anecdotal evidence, how to estimate the correct dosage of CBD for adults.

- If you are using CBD for a serious medical condition such as seizure disorders or inflammation from an autoimmune disorder, accurate CBD dosage is extremely important.

- For a healthy person who wants to take CBD as a nutritional bonus or supplement, dosing is not as critical.

- If you are taking your CBD in a hot drink such as coffee or tea, it is important to realize the milligram of the CBD will be greatly reduced because of the high temperature of the drink.

- CBD in low milligram dosage seems to be more of a stimulant for depression while CBD in higher dosages seems to be more of a sedative with anti-anxiety properties and sleep assistance.

It can be difficult figuring out a CBD dosage, FDA doesn't

regulate CBD, and there is no official recommended dosage.

The table below may help you with a starting dose based on body weight and the effects of CBD needed. These dosages are approximations and highly subjective due to the quality of CBD and the CBD company. Always consult your physician concerning the best starting dose before trying CBD for the first time, especially if you are on any medication as CBD may enhance or inhibit the potency of your medication.

Body Weight	Starting Dose	Low Dose	Medium Dose	High Dose
Under 100	5 mg	10 mg	20 mg	30 mg
100-110	10 mg	15 mg	25 mg	40 mg
111-130	15 mg	20 mg	30 mg	50 mg
131-150	20 mg	30 mg	40 mg	60 mg
151-170	30 mg	40 mg	50 mg	70 mg
171-190	40 mg	50 mg	60 mg	80 mg
191-210	50 mg	60 mg	70 mg	90 mg
211-230	60 mg	70 mg	80 mg	100 mg
231-250	70 mg	80 mg	90 mg	120 mg
251-300	80 mg	90 mg	110 mg	150 mg

Stronger doses than those listed may be more suitable for certain CBD consumers. These include people with severe pain or other debilitating symptoms, as well as those with a relatively high

CBD tolerance. CBD is not toxic and gradually increasing CBD dosage does not carry any known side effects and may increase the benefits of CBD.

The type of CBD product is also important to consider, since each one is associated with different concentrations, dosing methods, and effects. You will absorb a higher percentage of the CBD if taken sublingually. See chapter 13 for more details.

Dosage should begin small and increased with tolerability. Another thing to consider with dosage is the length of time CBD stays in the body. Multiple factors contribute including:

- Sex
- Weight
- Age
- Metabolism
- Lifestyle
- Frequency of use

Because of this, it can be very difficult to assess exactly how long CBD lingers in the body, and at what concentrations. CBD is fat-soluble and can build up and store in fat cells for quite a while, especially in a daily CBD user with a high-BMI (body-mass-index).

Those who live very active lifestyles, on the other hand, will most likely metabolize CBD at a faster rate than even a moderately active person. Likewise, all other things being equal, a younger person will metabolize CBD faster than someone much older.

How much and how often someone uses a CBD will have a major and perhaps the most significant effect on how long it takes for that CBD or any other supplement to dissipate completely.

Not a lot of research has been done on the safety and side effects of larger CBD doses but even in high doses like 1,500 milligrams per day, anecdotal evidence shows little to no side effects.

By following the suggested dosage on the CBD label or the chart above, and making certain the THC level is at zero or below 0.3% and the CBD is extracted from USA organically grown hemp, while considering the current completed research, you should be safe. If it appears you are having any reaction to the CBD, seek immediate medical attention.

Chapter Fifteen

The Next Step

Whether you are new to the world of CBD or you have been reading and researching for a time, I hope this book has cleared up a few questions and given you some direction as to stress causing symptoms and just how CBD can assist.

The next step is for you to consider how CBD might benefit you or someone you love. If you are leaning towards taking CBD, make certain you speak with a health care provider if you are pregnant, nursing, on any medication, under 18 or over 65 years old. CBD is amazing, but you need to make certain you start your CBD life on the right foot.

Furthermore, make sure you are purchasing a quality product and at a reasonable price. Don't be fooled by the extremely high price supplements as some companies mark CBD products up as high as 1000%. There is fake CBD selling for as little as $8. Look at the labs and thoroughly check out your source of CBD before making your first purchase.

Last, MaryAnn Stanger ND is only an email away. Please feel free to ask her any question. She usually respond within 48 hours.

ABOUT THE AUTHOR:

MaryAnn Stanger is a Naturopathic Doctor, Certified Digestive Health Specialist, Acupuncturist, Live Blood Analyst, NAET practitioner, Certified Aromatherapist, Author and has studied the Endocrine System extensively. She is a wife, mother of 8 and grandmother of 28.

In the early 90's, she decided to go back to school and learn all she could about health and nutrition. She wanted to be healthy. She wanted her family to be healthy. She wanted them to raise healthy children of their own. One goal was for her parents to live longer, healthier lives. So, she did it! She went back to school via distance learning with hands on applications and internships through Clayton College. It took her 7 years to complete, but she received her Naturopathic Doctors Degree in 1997. She then began a study of essential oils at Pacific Institute of Aromatherapy and became a certified Aromatherapist in 1998.

She created her own line of professional grade supplements in order to provide her patients and family the absolute highest quality products without fillers or additives, and at affordable prices. Zatural is based on her knowledge of natural synergies working in harmony to enhance the body towards health.

After discovering CBD and watching the effects it has on her life and the lives of those she served, she realized it may not be a cure-all, but it is a miracle. She formulated CBD synergies and added them to her Zatural line of supplements. She is excited to share with you the knowledge she has obtained and hopes it can bring stress-free relief to you or to those you love.

Contact information:

Customer Service: cs@zatural.com

Wholesale - info@zatural.com

Website: www.zatural.com

Phone - 208-969-1282

Clinical questions:

MaryAnn Stanger ND - nd@zatural.com

MaryAnn Stanger ND is the founder of Zatural. She also formulates all Zatural's supplements, CBD and skincare products.

Zatural uses only professional grade USA organic grown CBD.

All products are 3rd party tested for purity and accuracy of labeled content.

All Zatural products are manufactured at a GMP compliant facility located in Eden, Idaho.

Shipping is FREE to all USA address with low international shipping rates.

Wholesale and private label products are also available.